MEDICAL CANNABIS

A balanced, evidence based look
beyond the propaganda

MEREDITH
K.CONVERSE

MEDICAL CANNABIS : A Balanced, Evidence Based Look Beyond the Propaganda

Disclaimer Notice:

Please note the information contained within this document is for educational purposes only. Every attempt has been made to provide accurate, up to date, and reliable complete information no warranties of any kind are expressed or implied. Readers acknowledge that the author is not engaging in rendering legal, financial, or professional advice.

By reading any document, the reader agrees that under no circumstances are we responsible for any losses, direct or indirect, which are incurred as a result of use of the information contained within this document, including – but not limited to errors, omissions, or inaccuracies.

Also available on Amazon by the same author:
Probiotics: A Guide for Beginners
Create Wealth with the Principles of Feng Shui

Book and Cover design by Dee Cee

ISBN-13: 978-1500868932

First Edition: August 2014

CONTENTS

CONTENTS VI

INTRODUCTION 1

CHAPTER 1: THE HISTORY OF CANNABIS 9

CHAPTER 2: THE MEDICALIZATION OF CANNABIS 22

CHAPTER 3: MEDICAL USES FOR CANNABIS 37

CHAPTER 4: CANNABIS DELIVERY METHODS 54

CHAPTER 5: MEDICAL CANNABIS: POLITICS VS SCIENCE 67

CHAPTER 6: BIG BUSINESS AND MEDICAL CANNABIS 80

CHAPTER 7: THE CONCLUSION 88

ABOUT THE AUTHOR 94

Introduction

Cannabis is one of the hottest topics right now, in addition to being one of the most controversial. With the long, sordid history that this plant possesses, that should come as no surprise. While the recent trend of legalization in states like Washington and Colorado has muddled the argument, medical cannabis is still a reality in 23 States along with Washington DC. How did it get that way? Is it just a loophole to smoke recreational cannabis? Is there real science behind it? These are valid concerns that many have. The answers to them, however, aren't always clear. To remedy that, this book will cover every aspect of cannabis that is vital to the ongoing conversation.

For the vast majority of people, medical cannabis is still a mysterious topic. No matter how many people they might have met that have used cannabis in the past, the actual uses might be beyond their comprehension. The medical cannabis argument has two sides that are frequently at each other's throats, leaving very little to the casual observer. It is not an easy thing to understand without having clear-cut information. It doesn't have to always remain that way, no matter what the loudest advocates and opponents might say.

What Is It Exactly?

As an introduction to the medical cannabis argument, it is perhaps important to take a look at what cannabis actually is. There is a great deal of confusion over one aspect of it, although it is almost entirely shrouded in mystery to many people. The differences between the movements aiming to legalize hemp, medical cannabis, and recreational cannabis all have very different goals in mind, along with very different ways of achieving these goals. Each group typically has the opinion that they are the side that is right. This doesn't make the argument any easier to understand for most people.

Hemp

This book covers cannabis sativa, the variety of cannabis plants that contains THC. This distinction is crucial, due to the fact that it is very different from the cannabis plants that are used to create hemp. Hemp is one of the most versatile textile products in the world, although it has legal trouble as well. In the United States, it is legal to import and sell products manufactured with hemp, although it remains illegal to grow it. These strains have been bred specifically to reduce the THC levels and make it useless as a drug. The plant used to create the shoes and jewelry you wore in the 70s is not the same plant that is hailed as a miracle cure today. In fact, the use of hemp was something that was one of the most revolutionary textiles that the world has ever known. The magazine Popular Mechanics was actually preparing an in depth article covering the thousands of potential uses when it was banned. During the World War II effort, the government of the United States even asked people to grow hemp in order to help the war effort. They have since had a hard time coming to terms with this, but the fact remains that it is still illegal today and is the center of a great deal of controversy.

Medical Cannabis

Medical cannabis is the focus of this book, not the argument over hemp legalization or recreational use of cannabis. Medical cannabis has only been a recent development in comparison to recreational use, as far as western medicine is concerned. Many people claim that it is a miracle cure for everything from cancer to ADD/ADHD, while some say that it is nothing but the harmful, life-destroying drug that it has always been legally designated. This is the center of the argument discussed here. Which side is right? Are they both being entirely honest? The time has come to butt out the propaganda from both parties and get down to what should matter most to the public: the cold hard facts. This will not be simple, but it will make things clear.

Recreational Cannabis

Recreational cannabis involves the ingestion of cannabis sativa or cannabis indica, both containing large amounts of THC and other compounds known as CBD. Anyone living in America has most likely had some experience with this drastically different kind of cannabis, whether it is through contact with someone who has used it or used it themselves. The intoxicating effects have been the muse of musicians as well as the bane of addicts' existence.

For someone who used it in the Golden Age of San Francisco and hippie culture, there is a change that has taken place, which is worth describing here. The average THC content of DEA confiscated marijuana in the late 70s was around 1.4%, due to a variety of things such as long waits between harvest and consumer purchases and second rate grows in Mexico, while today it is estimated by the government agency that the average THC content is around 9%, with some reaching up to 37%. This is seen as bad news for at risk children, although it is also beneficial to marijuana advocates who point to the decrease in material required in joints, pipes, vaporizers, and "bongs." These will be covered more in depth in a later chapter.

This book contains an in depth look at all of these. In order to gain a greater understanding of what medical cannabis is, and what the future of it might be, it is vital that cannabis as a whole be understood. This includes the history of cannabis, how people ingest it, what it could be used to treat, what the political issues are, and what it could mean as a cash crop. The problem with discussing these is that both sides of the argument have large voices that want to be heard. The goal here is to break through that, finding the truth beneath the bias. In all, this coverage will touch on:

The History of Cannabis

Where did it come from? Who were the first users of cannabis? What started out as a medicine became a banned substance before finding life again. The 70s are over; however, the fight has started again in recent years. By looking at the history of cannabis dating back to the 3rd century BC, one can understand exactly what it has taken for cannabis to reach the current, modern age. It has not always been a clear-cut issue, as is obvious from the switches between wide spread acceptance and vehement suppression.

The Medicalization of Cannabis

The history of medical cannabis goes back farther than many assume, although it is a much more complicated than they assume as well. It did not start with the state of California in 1996 with the passing of their famous medical cannabis law. From the Chinese to the early 20th century, there have been uses covering a wide variety of conditions, carrying different levels of support in the medical community.

Medical Uses for Cannabis

A number of conditions are said to be alleviated by the use of cannabis, but research points to otherwise in many cases. This distinction is an important one, which is why looking at the scientific view and the mainstream view side by side is helpful.

Medical Cannabis: Politics vs. Science

With any medical issue, the politics can have a big impact on what is accepted. This is the case even when the scientific community is not in agreement. With medical cannabis, it often seems that legalization is driven more by politics than the research behind the potential benefits.

Big Business and Medical Cannabis

Considering the amount of money that can be made from cannabis, it should be no surprise that business owners and pharmaceutical companies alike are interested in joining the market. The dreadlocked dealers of the past are now being replaced by clean cut men in suits. Is this a good thing?

Cannabis Delivery Methods

There are lots of ways to take medical cannabis. Most people are familiar with smoking cannabis, but it can also be eaten in foods, taken as oil, vaporized, or taken as a prescription pill that contains an extract of the active ingredients. Of course, each method has its own advantages and disadvantages that can affect the choice of delivery for each individual patient. There is certainly a lot that goes into each of these topics, that much is for sure. By looking at each of them in a straightforward, balanced way, it is possible to understand what is happening in the medical cannabis movement, as well as where it might go.

Gaining a clear understand in this way is vital to the future of cannabis in a medical, economical, and political sense. The vast majority of people, especially those of older generations, can easily fall victim to the Cheerleaders on both sides of the argument. Advocates of complete legalization can often be found in the streets protesting political action and drawing a lot of attention to their cause. Medical cannabis patients also have a loud voice, one of the loudest, as they discuss what they say cannabis has done for them and what they would have to do without it. Finally, opponents of both options have the ability to control the argument in many cases. Political beliefs are often instilled in people during childhood, making it hard to change. With all of the obvious demonstrations, emotional talking points, and distorted facts and figures, the concept of an unbiased opinion goes out the window entirely.

An attempt will be made here to get through that. Research shows that no argument is clean, but there are obvious positions that can be backed up and some that should not play any part in your decision making process. Follow along and discover what the truth is, no matter what the propaganda tells you.

Chapter 1: The History of Cannabis

The history of cannabis as a plant is a very complex issue. In the last hundred years, the story has been filled with political fights and propaganda. Despite that, there is a very clear story that is important to anyone who wishes to understand the current fight. Many people may be surprised to learn that the history of cannabis didn't start with the widespread use during the Vietnam War. In fact, cannabis has a five thousand year history that extends far beyond many of the "traditional" medicines and products that most people think of.

Ancient China

The use of cannabis in ancient China is a topic that isn't discussed much when it comes to the recent medical marijuana movement. In reality, as far back as 2900 BC the Chinese Emperor Fu Hsi made mention of marijuana as a medicine. He stated that cannabis was a medicine that featured both yin and yang, an important aspect of Chinese culture. Over the next thousand years, cannabis turned up repeatedly in ancient writings. The Rh-Ya, a 15th century BC Chinese Pharmacopeia reference, cannabis was listed as a treatment for a variety of ailments. China was not the only place to discover cannabis in the old world, however, and it eventually spread through many eastern religions, including some that might surprise those who don't know much about the rich history of cannabis.

The Eastern World

Outside of China, people across the continent used cannabis in one way or another. Around 1200 BC, cannabis made it to Egypt. The Egyptians were known for being buried with important belongings and inside the tomb of Ramesses II there were containers of cannabis pollen. It is now known that they frequently prescribed it as a treatment for eye conditions and inflammation. In India, around 1000 BC, a drink known as Bhang was being used as an anesthetic. Bhang is made from combining cannabis with milk. As centuries went by, cannabis found more and more homes throughout that part of the world. From Muslim doctors using it as a herbal remedy to the use of hemp throughout the middle ages, different cultures certainly had different ways of looking at the cannabis plant and what the potential uses of it might be. In large part, cannabis was simply an everyday part of life throughout the eastern world for over two thousand years. While it may have not been the controversial topic that it is today when it was first introduced to America, it is no doubt the part of the story where the historical interest picks up in earnest.

Introduction to America

It seems hard to believe in the current political climate, but the cannabis plant was actually one of the first plants brought to America. The settlers at Jamestown in 1611 brought hemp fiber with them and it became a very important export. In fact, one of the first laws that was passed happened to be one requiring it be a crop in each settlers field. In the 18th century, cannabis plants were very common crops for the founding fathers. George Washington and Thomas Jefferson grew large crops of hemp at Mount Vernon and Monticello respectively. Throughout the 19th century, the world of cannabis was quiet. Towards the end of the century, however, the use had earned a reputation that started to affect the culture of the United States. The last two decades of the century saw marijuana becoming a very "fashionable narcotic." Hash shared space with oriental opium dens in the darker corners of the cities and it is believed that in New York City alone there were an estimated 500 hashish bars during the 1880s. Contrary to what politicians would say in the next century, these parlors were frequently visited by the white upper class citizens of the major cities.

The Beginning of Legal Action

At the start of the 20th century, the massive influx of cannabis users also brought a push for heavier legislative action. This is when many people point to a racial aspect of the laws surrounding cannabis, in part due to certain comments made by politicians at the time. The year was 1910 when a massive uprising in Mexico pushed a fresh wave of immigrants into the Southwestern United States. At the time, there was already a fear of certain immigrants, something that was always been an unfortunate side of American culture, although the Mexican immigrants brought something else with them: marijuana smoking. As they began coming into the country, police officers throughout Texas began making outlandish claims about cannabis and the kind of effects that it had on the people who used it. In particular, they claimed that it awakened a "lust for blood" and incited violent crimes throughout their state. These statements led to the rumor throughout the country that there were heavily intoxicated immigrants taking over who were spreading a "killer weed" that gave them superhuman strength. It was schoolchildren specifically who were claimed to be their targets.

At around the same time, sailors from the West Indies were bringing their own cannabis smoking practices into port cities in the Gulf of Mexico. Anyone who has ever been to New Orleans is familiar with the jazz music that inhabits it, but this was where much of it started. The sailors brought a drug with them that was a favorite among those musicians, but also African-Americans, prostitutes, and generally unsavory people. This led to a greater fear of "The Marijuana Menace" that was believed to be taking over. In particular, the propaganda focused on social deviants and inferior races as the culprits.

As time went on, the early drug warriors fought on. The tensions came to a head in 1937 with a man named Henry Anslinger. Anslinger was the US Narcotics Commissioner at the time and he began holding hearings in Congress that aimed to place federal restrictions on cannabis. Fueled by the paranoia that a film called "Reefer Madness" had started the year before, Anslinger lobbied for the Marihuana Tax Act. Reefer Madness started as a movie entitled "Tell Your Children" and was funded by a small church group as a way to scare the parents of children in the country. The film, in part, is what allowed Henry Anslinger to discuss that he had seen what "a small cannabis cigarette can do to one of our degenerate Spanish-speaking residents." Henry J Finger, a member of the State Board of Pharmacy in California, had also stated that immigrants were "initiating whites into this habit."

Anslinger's campaign against cannabis was greatly helped by the papers of William Randolph Hearst. Hearst used his papers to demonize the cannabis plant as a source of violent anger that must be stopped. Scholars argue that he was in fact trying to destroy the hemp industry. The hemp industry, at the time, could have potentially had the power to replace wood pulp paper used in the newspaper industry, which would have been a great loss to men like Hearst, Andrew Mellon, as well as the Du Pont family. Leading up to the hearings in Congress, Popular Mechanics was even preparing a story on the many uses of hemp and hailed it as one of the most useful fibers that the industrial world has ever known. This would effectively end that.

Despite the sparse evidence that men like these presented, and the poor attendance of the hearings as a whole, new laws were passed. The Marihuana Tax Act of 1937 placed a tax on physicians who were prescribing marijuana as well as pharmacists selling it. Effectively, this also made it illegal for anyone other than doctors to handle marijuana. They had the choice to pay the taxes on the marijuana they possessed, but this would also involve incriminating the person. It wasn't long before the first marijuana arrest was made in the United States under this law. On October 2, 1937, Samuel R Caldwell, a 58 year old unemployed laborer, was sentenced to four years of hard labor and a $1,000 fine. The proceeding decades were largely uneventful for marijuana action. The number of prescriptions for marijuana dropped dramatically immediately after the Marihuana Tax Act, a trend that was helped greatly by laws that came in the 1950s.

Severe Penalties

The era of severe penalties for marijuana began in earnest in 1951 with the Boggs Act. It turned out to be just the first of many moves like this that the federal government would make in an effort to get the marijuana menace under control. The Boggs Act established the very controversial mandatory minimum prison sentences for simple possession charges. Under this new law, it was possible to be sentenced to between two and five years in prison for first offenses. This was also the era in which addiction was seen as not only a disease, but a contagious one as well. It was also seen as incurable and many believed that these people simply had to be quarantined from the general public. This trend continued in terms of severe penalties. In 1956, only five years after the mandatory minimum sentences were established, cannabis was included in the Narcotics Control Act. This led to first-offense possession charges carrying up to ten years in prison with fines totaling up to $20,000.

The First Research

In the decade after cannabis was added to the Narcotics Control Act, cannabis began to see a resurgence in popularity, but earnest research also began to be done. The University of Mississippi brokered a deal with the federal government in 1968 to begin growing cannabis specifically for the purpose of research. The goal was to perform studies on preclinical toxicology in animals as well as clinical applications in humans. The next few years were contradictory for cannabis. The back and forth between the federal government and cannabis advocates was often hard to follow, due to what was seen as progressive research findings and backward legislative actions. 1970 brought the Controlled Substances Act that classified cannabis as a Schedule 1 narcotic, meaning it has "No Accepted Medical Use." That scheduling has been the source of controversy over the years, due to the fact that it is in the same category as psychedelics and heavy narcotics. At the time, Congress was asked if they agreed with this scheduling of marijuana. Their statement was as follows:

"Since there is still a considerable void in our knowledge of the plant and effects of the active drug contained in it, our recommendation is that marihuana be retained within schedule I at least until the completion of certain studies now underway to resolve the issue. If those studies make it appropriate for the Attorney General to change the placement of marihuana to a different schedule, he may do so in accordance with the authority provided under section 201 of the bill."

This implied that at a later date the scheduling would be changed if research showed that it should be altered. Ever since this action, people have come back time and time again pointing to this promise being unfulfilled. Whenever a movement is made to have cannabis rescheduled, the government is forced to explain how their opinion has changed since this time. In the meantime, NORML was founded, which is the National Organization for the Reform of Marijuana Laws. This organization has existed since 1970 as an advocate of marijuana and they have been at the forefront of the fight.

The research that was being performed was short lived, however, as President Richard Nixon refused to legalize cannabis after a recommendation from the Shafer Commission. His response was:

"As you know, there is a Commission that is supposed to make recommendations to me about this subject; in this instance, however, I have such strong views that I will express them. I am against legalizing marijuana. Even if the Commission does recommend that it be legalized, I will not follow that recommendation... I can see no social or moral justification whatever for legalizing marijuana. I think it would be exactly the wrong step. It would simply encourage more and more of our young people to start down the long, dismal road that leads to hard drugs and eventually self-destruction."

The Shafer Commission was put together as a bipartisan group that was charged with determining if personal use should be decriminalized throughout the country. Their findings that cannabis should be decriminalized were largely swept under the rug by President Nixon. Following the findings and his refusal, he announced the War on Drugs on June 17, 1971. This effectively began all out war on cannabis and the people using it, although cannabis went on to find more popularity than ever in the coming years.

The Push for Legalization

Cannabis found a new home with millions of Americans throughout the 1960s. That trend continued through the seventies, even though drug laws became stricter. In the times of Jimmy Carter's Presidency, cannabis was incredibly popular. Carter himself worked to decriminalize cannabis, although eleven states did so on their own throughout the decade. Interestingly enough, President Carter would later sign a letter alongside Bush and Ford saying that states should not decriminalize cannabis, showing how the tides can change when it comes to medical cannabis. Throughout the 1980s, no legislation was passed that had a major effect on legalization. In 1989 there was a ruling saying that it should be rescheduled, although the DEA overruled it.

As the 1990s rolled on, however, several discoveries were made when it comes to cannabis. This would mark the beginning of the second wave of medical cannabis research. In just a few years medical cannabis would change forever in the state of California, but the research was just beginning to kick into high gear. 1992 brought the discovery of the first endocannabinoid. This is the brain's natural version of THC, which is released with strenuous exercise. When this was discovered, it made it possible to take an in depth look at the kinds of things that cannabis does to the brain, in addition to studying whether or not there are any other chemicals that have a similar effect.

Three years later, another attempt was made at rescheduling cannabis. The second petition to have it rescheduled was filed in July by the National Director of the National

Organization for the Reform of Marijuana Laws. In January of 1997, a similar complaint was filed. This time it came from the New England Journal of Medicine. Their editorial stated that it should be up to physicians and patients to decide if it had medical value. More successful efforts to enact medical cannabis happened throughout the 1990s, but that will be saved for the next chapter. At present there are 23 states that have legalized medical cannabis, in addition to Washington DC. It is expected that there will be many more in the next election cycle coming in 2016. Even more recently, Colorado and Washington have legalized recreational cannabis as well in landmark votes in 2012. Much like the medical cannabis motions expected to be on ballots in the next election cycle, several states that already have medical cannabis are expected to have recreational initiatives on the ballot.

The Future

The history of cannabis is certainly an interesting topic. Cultures all across the world have had cannabis as a part of their culture at one time or another, whether it was as a national treat or as an illegal substance that is looked down upon. That eclectic history is what makes the future exciting as well for those in the medical cannabis movement. While the scientific community is not as fast moving as advocates would like, this is surely a topic that isn't going to go away any time soon. That is especially true given the fact that there are already more states looking at putting legalization efforts on the ballot. The excitement that people on both sides have makes it something that is worth following into the future. It can be easy to get lost in the day to day news happenings, but at the very least a casual observer can see that the past and present are only the beginning for this interesting plant.

Chapter 2: The Medicalization of Cannabis

Cannabis has a history of medicalization that has been in high gear primarily since the 1950s. There were medical uses for much farther back, but in the United States it has been a particularly hot topic over the past 60 years. For thousands of years it was a staple of Indian and Asian medicine before being introduced to the west in the middle of the 19th century. It was soon taken up enthusiastically by doctors across Europe and the United States, until it found itself on the other side of the law at a certain point.

Throughout the entire history of cannabis, it has meant a lot of different things to a lot of different people. Some see it as a harmless recreational pastime, while some think it is a cure all for almost any disease on the face of the planet. The history of it as a medicine started long before the day that any of the actual chemicals inside it had ever been isolated, or even before it was understood as something that had any active chemicals in it.

Ancient Medicine

In the ancient world, medical cannabis was a particularly popular topic. Hemp was used in Taiwan as far back as 10,000 years ago, although the Chinese are believed to be the source of it as a medical treatment. One of the early emperors of China, Shen-Nung, also happened to be a pharmacologist. He wrote a book on medical treatments that included cannabis as treatments for a large variety of ailments including gout, rheumatism, and constipation. Many years later, Hua Tuo began using it as an anesthetic in China as well. In his case, he would mix a powdered form with wine before administering it.

Over the years in China, more and more people recommended it as a source of medication. In a compendium of Chinese medicine, cannabis is listed as one of the fifty fundamental herbs in traditional Chinese medicine. In that book, cannabis was described as having 120 different treatments for diseases. According to *Chinese Materia Medica: Vegetable Kingdom:*

> "Every part of the hemp plant is used in medicine ... The flowers are recommended in the 120

different forms of disease, in menstrual disorders, and in wounds. The achenia, which are considered poisonous, stimulate the nervous system, and if used in excess, will produce hallucinations and staggering gait. They are prescribed in nervous disorders, especially those marked by local anesthesia.

The seeds ... are considered to be tonic, demulcent, alterative, laxative, emmenagogue, diuretic, anthelmintic, and corrective. They are prescribed internally in fluxes, post-partum difficulties, aconite poisoning, vermillion poisoning, constipation, and obstinate vomiting. Externally they are used for eruptions, ulcers, favus, wounds, and falling of the hair.

The oil is used for falling hair, sulfur poisoning, and dryness of the throat. The leaves are considered poisonous, and the freshly expressed juice is used as an anthelmintic, in scorpion stings, to stop the hair from falling out and to prevent it from turning gray. ... The stalk, or its bark, is considered to be diuretic ... The juice of the root is ... thought to have a beneficial action in retained placenta and post-partum hemorrhage. An infusion of hemp ... is used as a demulcent drink for quenching thirst and relieving fluxes."

This incredibly long list of uses is something that may not have stood up to modern medicine, but China certainly found it incredibly useful. In terms of ancient medicine, this could actually be seen as a very progressive and effective treatment, even though now we have things that are much more effective and carry far fewer side effects. As a part of the ancient medicinal world, China had a very important role in deciding what was popular. They are not the only culture to take advantage of the medicinal power, though.

Ancient Egypt

Although it was touched on above, ancient Egypt had many different uses for cannabis as a medical treatment. The Ramesseium III Papyrus, the Berlin Papyrus, and the Chester Beatty Medical Papyrus VI all talk about the kinds of uses that it had, including relieving pain from hemorrhoids and more.

The West

In the colonies, it was used as a way to cure cholera's vomiting, the muscle spasms of rabies, a sedative, and an antibiotic. There were still problems, however, as for a long time it was hard to use as medicine due to the fact that it wasn't water soluble. This caused it to be useless in the world of hypodermic syringes as they came into wider use. That did not stop it from eventually catching on as medicine.

Throughout the 19th century, the use began to grow, even though there was scant research on it. Based only on anecdotal evidence, there were over 2000 cannabis medicines by the late 1930s. After the passing of the Marihuana Tax Act, however, the number of prescriptions dropped dramatically and it eventually went back into obscurity.

The Resurgence

As the United States entered the 1960s, however, cannabis once again became an incredibly popular drug of choice for millions of people in America. At the same time, the scientific community became once again interested in taking a looking at what potential uses it could have. The research that happened throughout the later years of the 60s and into the early years of the 70s was incredibly fast paced. This is considered the first wave of proper research into the topic, although it was long after the initial uses of medical cannabis. At the time, it was more of an effort to understand whether or not cannabis should be decriminalized, however, rather than understanding every benefit that it could provide the human body. There was very little clinical research published at the time. The goal of proving that something is NOT harmful is a difficult task and many scientists were simply not up to the task. Based on the research that they did do, however, they did not find any specific reasons that cannabis should have stayed illegal. This was largely unnoticed, however, by the legislative bodies. Running side by side with this newer interest in cannabis as a medicine was a stronger push towards legislative action. In the 1970s, stricter and stricter laws were put in place that regulated cannabis and the kind of research that could be done on it.

Several conferences took place during this time that illustrated the negative effects that cannabis had, rather than the potential clinical applications. The quasi-toxicological work left many with the notion that it was a deadly compound that should remain illegal.

The people who were taking part in these conferences had already made up their mind, although there were still scientists arguing that the verdict wasn't yet in. One of the problems at this same time was that there had been virtually no research funded by government grants that looked into the topic. Despite that, there was research going on through the 1970s in other countries. One of their goals was to isolate THC as an active compound in cannabis. Not only that, the goal was to decide if THC was actually biologically responsible for the effects that people were experiencing.

In order to study that, scientists at Oxford set out to isolate it and study the effects. This research was all funded, it is worth pointing out, without government help. It came much later, but the initial research was done without the help that many medical researchers have. Scientists credit the discovery of the receptor that is affected by THC with saving their research all together. Without that discovery, they believe that it would have gone the way of alcohol and only ever be studied in terms of negative effects. One researcher said that if that discovery had not been made, there would merely be a handful of scientists around the world puttering around, but not doing earnest research that would have ever been conclusive.

Abuse Clouds Research

While THC was being isolated for the first time, there was also a great deal of recreational cannabis use that was getting much more attention than the scientific research that was going on. Tinctures of cannabis were already banned by the early 1970s, but research continued to be pushed to only show negative effects that the community wanted to be confirmed. That tincture was a huge loss for the pharmacological world due to the fact that it was the primary source of cannabinoids for researchers.

The Return to Research

Research found a way to continue, at least in animal trials. There were no receptors discovered in the brain at the time, so all that could be done was descriptive work for the most part. Those years were largely filled with observing animals after being given cannabis extracts. The animals were seen as behaving normally for a while, before going into a trance-like state, which is apparent to anyone that has ever used cannabis before in a recreational way. What remained a problem was that there was no known receptor inside of the brain that could be observed under exposure to cannabis. The THC could have only been one of many chemicals that act on the same part of the brain, but there was no way of knowing. Towards the later years of the 1970s, chemicals like cocaine and amphetamines had been getting a lot of attention in the scientific world, with cannabis largely on the backburner.

The Synthetic Solution

Fortunately, the introduction of a new synthetic THC analogue brought on the ability to kick research back into high gear and understand what was going on. With the introduction of Nabilone in 1981, Eli Lilly created a synthetic cannabinoid that could be studied. Marinol followed closely after in 1985. Nabilone in particular was found to be moderately effective in alleviating the symptoms of fibromyalgia. It has also been tested for Parkinson's, MS, nausea from chemotherapy, inflammatory bowel disease, and many more. Combining these synthetic compounds with the discovery of the endocannabinoids was a very powerful tool for medical cannabis researchers. Researchers could now identify specific reactions inside of the brain and study the effects of CBD and THC in depth, without having to rely on actual raw cannabis products.

Scientists Get Organized

By the 1990s, there were a lot of reports coming out showing that people had been self-medicating with cannabis for a variety of disorders. With this out in the open, there was a great deal more interest in researching the clinical aspects. In response to that resurgence in popularity, the International Cannabinoid Research Society was established. It had until that point been difficult to communicate with other people who were doing medical cannabis research, but this organization changed all of that.

Once again, the problem came up that it was almost impossible to have any kind of plant extract used as medicine or for research purposes. As the early 1990s carried on, however, more and more MS patients in particular were pushing for cannabis plant extracts to be available for treating their symptoms. The primary concern was that it still wasn't entirely understood if cannabis was a medication or if there were only certain elements that were therapeutic. That is why medical cannabis was approved in the state of California in 1996. This law made it legal for primary caregivers to prescribe cannabis as a treatment for a variety of disorders. Patients have the ability to purchase the cannabis from designated dispensaries or grow a limited amount of it for their own personal use.

As medical cannabis became a reality in other states as well, the use of opioids and NSAIDs dramatically dropped. This was due in large part to many pain management patients making the switch to medical cannabis. This led to more research being done in a clinical setting. Nabilone was studied with this in mind throughout the 1990s, looking at patients that had been unable to find any relief from their chronic pain problems. In the early studies on pain relief from Nabilone, nearly one third of all patients reported having marked relief from use of the drug compared to the chemical compounds that they had been prescribed in the past. In every case, even those who said that they were not helped by the drug said that they preferred taking it to taking other painkillers. This was an exciting development for the scientific world when it comes to cannabis. Larger trials were scheduled, although scientists still weren't sure exactly what was going to happen when people were prescribed these drugs on a long term basis.

The New Millennium

The year 2000 brought research into cannabis that had previously been unmatched. At the same time that a study was being performed at James Paget Hospital, there were pieces of research being undertaken at Oxford as well. The patients that were studied in both cases were seen as being at the end of the line in terms of treatment options. In the year that followed, definitive, randomized controlled trials began that reflected the same kind of findings that scientists had seen in the past. What stood out to the researchers were the relatively few side effects that people experienced compared to the benefits they received. With drugs like morphine patients were often left in far more of a haze than with the synthetic cannabinoid drugs that they were being given as a part of these trials.

Even these trials were marked with skepticism, however, due to the fact that an ever growing part of the population was reporting that smoking cannabis was helping with their chronic pain. The image of a dreadlocked college student discussing their chronic pain is not very convincing. That same skepticism is what has driven research since. A focus on empirical data has been important to researchers who have wanted to sincerely find an answer, rather than those who only want to prove that cannabis is harmful.

The major study that looked at the results people had with smoking cannabis asked 4,500 people to fill out a 70-question form that would assess every aspect of their cannabis use and the kind of results that they had. The questionnaire covered where the people found their cannabis, what type of cannabis it was, how they felt after using it, what made them take more or less, and more. During this time, some researchers began to understand that patients can in fact be trusted with their own dosage.

Throughout the 90s, more and more doctors were allowing their patients to dose their own morphine after surgery. There was no way to know for sure how much pain medication a patient needed, but the patient would know if they were still in pain. By listening to patients in this same way, doctors were able to begin understanding the medical cannabis issue in a way that had previously been impossible.

The Effects on Children

It became evident after the pain management studies that there were large groups of children that had been unable to find a solution for the nausea and vomiting associated with chemotherapy. This has been a controversial topic in the years since, but the fact remains that children have a particularly hard time dealing with certain types of illnesses and cannabis has shown a possible benefit to them in this way. The study looked at a group of children who were aged from one to thirteen years of age. The children were given THC under the tongue in varying doses and not one child ever reported nausea again after the application. This was a breakthrough study, although the act of giving THC to children has been met with quite a bit of adversity.

Since the time that those studies were done, at the beginning of the 21st century, the medicalization of cannabis has in large part taken a turn for being patient driven. The most recent trials have shared the focus on children that the last study discussed did. Charlotte's Web was the strain of cannabis specifically designed to have the potential to be used in children suffering from a certain kind of epilepsy that has so far been largely untreatable in many cases. This has brought even more controversy to the table, with many people even uprooting their families to travel to medical cannabis states in order to get the kind of treatment that they see as the only option available to them at this point in their disease.

Despite the medical advancements that have been made in this century alone, many people are still finding that they do not tolerate pharmaceutical drugs very well. After growing increasingly tired and jaded with modern medicine, it is only logical that people would start to look elsewhere. The dramatic side effects of some prescription drugs can be worse than the condition that they are attempting to treat. This is a point of contention for the medical community, but it is nonetheless an important piece of anecdotal evidence. The activism that this has spurred has brought more and more people into clinical trials studying the topic of cannabis as medicine. This has recently applied to elderly people who might not have been a part of the hippie culture, but found out about the potential benefits from their children and are now increasingly interested in learning if it will work for them.

The Medicalization of Cannabis

The history of cannabis in terms of medical treatment has been a long and interesting journey. It certainly has picked up in the past few decades, although it isn't likely to end here. The future of the medical cannabis movement is largely being driven by patients and politics rather than science in large part, although it doesn't discount the work of the hard working scientists that have been described here. The researchers that performed the studies described in this chapter have been charged with an almost impossible task, although they have persevered and taken up the charge.

After understanding the history of medical cannabis specifically, it is now time to understand the medical uses for cannabis that have been brought to the public's eye in the past few years. There are two distinct viewpoints on this topic: the mainstream viewpoint and the view of the scientific community. As evident in this chapter, the scientific community is not against the idea, but it is important to keep things in perspective when judging a topic that has such a large impact on the public at large.

Chapter 3: Medical Uses for Cannabis

Medical cannabis has been hailed as a miracle cure for an increasingly large number of medical problems. People using cannabis have claimed that it helps them with almost any health issue they are having, whether physical or mental, although the actual scientific research behind many of these can be optimistic at best. The problem with the legality of medical cannabis is that it is often illegal to perform any kind of research that is capable of confirming what has been said about it. That hasn't stopped anecdotal evidence from largely deciding what kinds of medical cannabis treatments are suitable. This chapter will provide a look at the most talked about treatments of medical cannabis. There are dozens of conditions that medical cannabis has been linked to, but there are a few that stand out among the rest. The twenty two year old claiming that cannabis cured their ADD may not be very believable, although science has worked hard to provide a more substantial understanding of these conditions and treatments.

The Mainstream View

The mainstream view of the benefits of medical cannabis has largely been driven by a political movement that it can treat almost any disorder known to man. It has been hailed as a near-panacea for conditions ranging from simply chemotherapy-induced nausea to actually curing cancer. The support for medical cannabis on a mainstream level is certainly very passionate. The majority of people polled on medical cannabis believe that it has a very beneficial purpose not only as an addition to other forms of treatments, but also as a complete replacement for many traditional forms of medicine.

In general, cannabis is increasingly being seen as a completely harmless plant. Many people agree that it has no negative effect on the lungs or at the very least that it is less harmful than cigarettes. There is also the belief that it is great for "self-medicating" conditions that are problematic. Things like pain, depression, ADD/ADHD, and more are touted as easily cured by simply smoking a little bit of weed from time to time. The reason for this is very simple. Look at what works best in a political campaign. Medical cannabis advocates have very emotional stories and very effective ways of presenting patients that have benefited from medical cannabis. This is not to say that there is no evidence for the benefits of medical cannabis. The sentiment of the mainstream view is largely sincere and is in tune with the general distrust of medications as a whole. The move towards herbalism and natural remedies for disorders has been growing at an exponential speed in recent years. Twenty years ago this would have been unheard of.

The mainstream view of cannabis has drastically changed since it was made legal in the state of California back in 1996. Millions of people are now in support of its use for a number of disorders, most prominently HIV/AIDS patients, chemotherapy patients, and those with MS. This change in climate has been an interesting one. Take the case of a psychiatry professor by the name of Lester Grinspoon. This professor was someone that started out with a bias towards hoping to discover the harmful effects that cannabis was having on the public at large. Over time, his position changed greatly as his son found it helped with his chemotherapy. It was then that he began doing research that was much like the discovery that the general public has had when it comes to medical cannabis.

In the 1970s, it was considered political suicide to discuss cannabis in any capacity other than making the laws governing it stricter than ever. In the past year, however, it has become a hot topic that can push a politician to power in some cases. There are very few things that get democrats to the polls more than the potential passing of a medical cannabis bill. In the past year alone, several high profile politicians have come out in support of medical cannabis in ways that would have previously been very unlikely to say the least. The Democratic Governor of Missouri, Jay Nixon, was recently asked about medical cannabis and he said that he is rejecting recreational cannabis flat out, but that he would be open to the idea of medicinal cannabis if it was an agreement between state legislators and the medical community.

Similarly, Louisiana Governor Bobby Jindal, a staunch Republican, has even come on to the side of medical cannabis. Gov Jindal said that he would also be against legalizing recreational cannabis, but that for legitimate patients medical cannabis is an option that he is open to in his state. This has been echoed across the country. Senator Harry Reid put it this way, "If you'd asked me this question a dozen years ago, it would have been easy to answer- I would have said no, because cannabis leads to other stuff. But I can't say that anymore." When Nixon first established the

War on Drugs it was to root out the communists and the degenerates that were using cannabis, something that many people in the public agreed with. They saw the kinds of people that were using it openly and associated some of their behavior with all users, even though they likely knew many more people who were using it in private.

A prime example on how the mainstream view of medical cannabis affects laws is in the case of Ed Rosenthal. This man had been arrested and charged with growing cannabis. During his trial, the medical aspect did not come up a single time. He was simply tried as a criminal who was growing an illegal substance, rather than focusing on the healing properties he believed he was providing. After the case was over, jurors were asked about this particular aspect of the trial and they were shocked to discover that he was using the plant as medicine. Had they known that, they said, they would have had a much different opinion of the case as a whole. These kinds of stories greatly affect the public opinion on cannabis. It is up to the public to decide what kinds of laws are passed, but only knowing certain bits of information makes them fallible as well. This is not to say that their opinion doesn't matter, but it is worth pointing out that there is a lot of research that needs to be done before anyone can make up their mind once and for all.

Science Based Medicine

Science based medicine has a much different view of medical cannabis. That is not to say that science believes there is absolutely no place for cannabis in medicine. No matter how hard a doctor fought against the drug warriors of the Summer of Love, at this point they will concede that there is some benefit, although they will disagree over how effective cannabis is or what it can medically be used to treat. The scientific world views cannabis as something that has been promoted more by the mainstream view than by their own. There is a large disconnect when it comes to the kinds of things that medical science has proven to be effective and the kinds of things that cannabis is hailed as a cure for.

In many cases, the results of studies done on cannabis have been greatly exaggerated. The studies have indeed discovered potential medical benefits, but how effective that connection is has not been established by the scientific community. The connection is something that the scientific community would like to look at more in depth. The problem comes in the form of the general difficulty in being allowed to perform research. In order for a group to begin a study, they will have to register with the Drug Enforcement Agency, submit a special application to the Food and Drug Administration, and gain access to cannabis from the

National Institute on Drug Abuse. All of that can only happen in places where they are allowed to even begin the process. Given that difficulty, many have given up on researching cannabis as a whole.

The scientific view of cannabis has now turned to specific compounds inside of the plant. The most well performed and regarded studies have been conducted using purified cannabinoids. With that in mind, it is easy to see why the scientific community is often skeptical of claims about medical cannabis. They have not studied smokable or edible forms of marijuana enough to make a confident decision.

One thing that must be included in this section is the problem of research that is meant to only discredit cannabis, not prove that it is actually effective at treating any kind of disorders. A complaint that has been raised repeatedly by scientists is that they have been tasked with deciding whether or not cannabis should be decriminalized, but they are asked to verify a negative, which they cannot do. In some cases, they have even been asked specifically to study the harmful effects, rather than simply compile unbiased data that can be used to make decisions. That is not the case with all scientific research, of course. Otherwise, there would not be any positive conclusions like the ones that have been seen.

It is something to be wary of, however, especially as time moves forward and more research is allowed to take place in states where not only medical, but also recreational cannabis has been legalized.

The Common Uses

There are hundreds of uses for medical cannabis according to some people. In the early days of its use in the United States, there were sometimes 300 different cannabis medications available. Today, however, there are only a few common uses that have been able to stand up to scientific reasoning, if not always remarkably well.

Nausea

Nausea, in particular nausea that is associated with chemotherapy, can be something that severely inhibits a person's ability to carry on their everyday life. During chemotherapy, nausea and vomiting make it almost impossible to eat, which leads to dramatic weight loss that impairs the body's ability to fight of the cancer that the chemo is trying to beat. Anecdotal evidence from hundreds of chemotherapy patients shows that cannabis can be an effective way of treating the nausea and vomiting most commonly associated with the treatment. In some cases, this is the only way of treating the nausea. Doctors across the world have noticed that their patients, when using medical cannabis, have noticeably less side effects and respond much better to the chemotherapy.

On the other side of the argument, scientists are concerned that cannabis can't meet the needs of patients who are deep in chemotherapy treatments. John Glaspy from the University of California at Los Angeles has stated that "medical cannabis has some effect on nausea and vomiting, but it is a weak effect, and it doesn't compete well with the targeted drugs that have been developed." This sentiment has been shared by many other researchers that have found the minor effect that medical cannabis has on nausea doesn't work well enough to replace the existing medications that chemotherapy patients have used for many years now.

Glaucoma

Glaucoma is perhaps one of the most well known disorders that is treated by medical cannabis. When it comes to jokes about red eyes and cannabis possession, glaucoma is the go-to joke many people have on hand. Dating back to the 1970s it has been understood that cannabis could help treat this condition that leads to progressive nerve damage in the eyes that can eventually lead to blindness. The original studies that were done on this particular topic found that it could dramatically reduce the pressure inside of the eyes. This is effectively the only way to treat glaucoma, whether accomplished with medical cannabis or another prescription drug. There is a problem in that the cannabis has been found to be a very suitable treatment, but it only works for around four hours at a time. As should probably be evident, this means that patients will have to use the cannabis several times a day, which can be a problem if they are smoking it. This is a condition that requires twenty-four hours a day pressure relief in order to effectively stop future damage that could end in blindness. This means that patients will have to take into account the other side effects of cannabis. In some cases, it will be necessary to use large amounts several times a day, which can leave many people feeling incredibly intoxicated and unable to function throughout their daily life.

Pain Management

Chronic pain can get in the way of living life for millions of people across the world. There are a lot of different ways people can end up with these kinds of chronic pain problems, but no matter how the patient ended up with the pain, dealing with it is always a struggle. Study after study has shown that medical cannabis can be a powerful tool for managing chronic pain. There are two sides to the findings that have shown this. The first is that cannabis can act as a mild pain reliever in the same vein as codeine. It has also been found that it can enhance the effects of opiate pain killers, allowing them to be dosed in much smaller amounts. There are, however, some concerns about the use of medical cannabis as a way of managing pain. The criticism is that there is no analgesic property specifically tied to cannabis. The short term CNS euphoria can be very helpful, but it might not be the best choice for long term pain relief. Overall, cannabis is seen as a potentially effective painkiller, but it should not be the first line of attack since there are better-tolerated medications on the market.

Appetite Stimulation

Anyone that has smoked cannabis knows about the "munchies" that typically come along with the euphoria. It has been the source of jokes in movies over the decades. This appetite stimulation could have very helpful effects for people who suffer from diseases like cancer or HIV/AIDS. People with these diseases frequently suffer from what is known as cachexia, or "wasting." This kind of wasting problem can easily be solved by smoking cannabis. The problem is that this is an issue that has other solutions as well. Research has not been conclusive as to the long-term efficacy, however. Much like the original research into cannabis, it is often a difficult task of understanding whether or not it is a specific compound in the cannabis that is causing this effect or if it is not something that a company would be able to synthesize and obtain the same effects without the use of a drug.

Multiple Sclerosis

Multiple Sclerosis, or MS, is one of the most debilitating neurological disorders that people face in the modern world. This disorder is an inflammatory disease and causes the insulation of the nerve cells inside of the brain and spinal cord to become damaged. This causes the nervous system to lose the ability to communicate, which leads to a variety of physical, mental, and psychiatric problems. Montel Williams is perhaps the most famous advocate of medical cannabis for the treatment of MS. He has long been a supporter and credits cannabis with providing relief that allows him to function on a daily basis. Many other MS patients have echoed this benefit and claim that it is responsible for their ability to live their life.

A study of 100 patients suffering from multiple sclerosis was performed, which looked at the results that they had when using a spray or pill form of cannabis, rather than smoked. The findings showed that forms of cannabis that are anything other than smoked are not efficient at alleviating the involuntary muscle movements. Conclusions were problematic as well because many of the benefits that patients reported could not be verified by the doctors and scientists that were performing the study. This suggests that more testing is necessary before it can be reasonably prescribed to patients with confidence.

Epileptic Seizures

One condition that has gained a great deal of exposure over the past few years has been children with epileptic seizures, a condition known as Dravet Syndrome. Sanjay Gupta's CNN documentary "Weed" covered the story of a young girl named Charlotte Figi, who has up to 300 seizures every single week. After a variety of other medical treatments, they turned to medical cannabis. This kind of story has been echoed time and time again throughout the country, although there is still the problem of figuring out what kind of long term effects this treatment might have. According to medical cannabis advocates, the high cannabidiol and low THC strains of cannabis used in creating cannabis oils deliver the proper active chemicals that have beneficial effects for Dravet's syndrome, without any of the accompanying high that is typical of cannabis. The medical journal *Epilepsia* has detailed a series of articles on the topic, many of them pointing to beneficial effects. A study found that both THC and CBD have the potential to display anti-convulsive properties when tested on animals. In human beings, similar effects have been noticed. The problem for opponents of medical cannabis is that there is a severe lack of double-blind randomized studies illustrating this same kind of treatment's success. There have not been any randomized studies on epileptic groups, although they are in the planning stages and will hopefully begin in the coming year.

Yet another concern for those on both sides of the argument is the worry that when medical cannabis is given to epileptic patients it can sometimes lead to symptoms such as anxiety, schizophrenia, or even addiction. Until much more extensive research has been completed on the topic, this will remain something that is speculated and it will continue to be a cause for concern.

Cancer

Cancer is a deadly disorder and one that many people lose their battle with. In terms of medical cannabis, it is perhaps one of the most well researched diseases. Compared to things like depression and nausea, cancer has been studied in depth and there are measurable results that have shown that medical cannabis can be very effective. There are, of course, still concerns that many people have.

Brain Cancer

Studies published in the British Journal of Cancer, The Journal of Neuroscience, and The Journal of Pharmacology and Experimental Therapeutics have all stated that THC could have beneficial effects. The first study found that brain tumor cells were decreased in some cases, but in most it was at least slowed. The anti-tumor effects of THC and CBD have both been found to work well in some patients.

Breast Cancer

Breast cancer is an increasing problem in the female population and medical cannabis is now being researched as a way of increasing the effectiveness of treatment in addition to traditional cancer drugs. The US National Library of Medicine published a study that found cannabidiol significantly inhibits breast cancer proliferation and it can drastically reduce the size of the tumors.

Lung Cancer

Lung cancer is a worry for people who use cannabis in the first place, but research from Harvard has found that medical cannabis could actually be used for treatment of certain types of lung cancer. Two Harvard Medical School studies have found that THC and CBD can help shrink lung cancer cells and prevent further growth.

Other conditions that cannabis is believed to treat include:

- Anxiety
- PTSD
- Brain recovery after a stroke
- Diabetes
- Repairing damage done to lungs by tobacco smoke
- Stop progression of Alzheimer's disease
- Control muscle spasms
- Aid treatment for Hepatitis C
- Control inflammatory bowel diseases
- Aid in weight loss
- Improve symptoms of lupus
- Eliminate Crohn's disease
- Many, many more

These medical conditions are often hailed as the only option for some people, but that doesn't mean there isn't any truth to them.

The Mainstream World vs. the Science World

One of the important things to understand with medical cannabis is that some of the conditions that are supposed to be "treated" are actually simply side effects of the euphoria that cannabis provides. This is not to downplay the alleviation of depression, for example, although other medications could potentially be much more helpful without having the other side effects of cannabis, or requiring extended use on a daily basis in order to achieve the desired effects. As time passes, there is a greater chance that researchers will be able to better understand the kinds of things that medical cannabis can treat. At the end of the day, there simply isn't enough data at the moment. In the future, there is a very good possibility that science could discover that it is highly effective for a large number of conditions. With that being said, the mainstream view may continue to rule the argument, even if the scientific world hasn't reached that point yet.

Chapter 4: Cannabis Delivery Methods

There are many different ways that medical cannabis patients, and everyday users, ingest their cannabis. Smoking cannabis is iconic. It is what the vast majority of people think of when they picture cannabis. Memories of Woodstock come floating back. The smell of pot smoke filling the air. In the modern world, however, that isn't the only option. It is an especially poor choice for people sick with cancer or other serious illnesses. In these cases, it is important to look at other delivery methods.

There are five primary ways that people deliver the active ingredients of marijuana into their system. Depending on what condition a person has, they might choose to begin:

- Smoking Cannabis
- Vaporizing Cannabis
- Eating Cannabis
- Using Cannabis Oils
- Taking Prescription Cannabis Pills

The Importance of Delivery

The way that people ingest cannabis has a large impact on the kind of results that they have, but it also plays a large role in the side effects that patients experience as a result of using cannabis. There are many who say that no health problems can come from ingesting cannabis, but the fact of the matter is that there certainly are. Granted, some of those negative effects come from the particular way that they are taking it in, rather than from the actual plant matter itself. That is why this chapter will cover the variety of methods that are most commonly used throughout the world of medical cannabis and beyond.

Smoking Cannabis

Smoking cannabis is no doubt the most common form of delivery. When it comes to the everyday users, rolling a joint or lighting a pipe is by far the most tried and true method that they stand by. Many users find that they smoke cannabis throughout their entire life and never try any of the other delivery methods. Even though people have been smoking cannabis in hopes of gaining the desired effects for some time, it is hard to imagine a less efficient way of taking something that is meant to be a medication. There has been a great deal of research done on cannabis smoke and the effect that it has on the human body, though. It has been found time and time again that cannabis smoke is far less harmful and less carcinogenic than tobacco smoke. That being said, cannabis smoke is also inhaled without a filter, giving it the opportunity to deposit up to four times the amount of tar that cigarette smoke does. This also means it has the same ability to irritate the respiratory system in other ways as well. That is, of course, something that is highly argued and usually met with a lot of contention. Research is still ongoing to attempt to reach the final say on the topic, however. With regular, moderate use, however, it doesn't appear to have a dramatic effect on lung function. This is based on users who smoke one joint a day for up to seven years. The problem with this is that many patients who would use medical cannabis would be forced to smoke it four to five times a day in order to get all day relief from their ailments.

The fact remains that it is simply not the best designed method of delivering a medicine to a patient. Burning plant matter and inhaling the hundreds of byproducts of that it creates might deliver THC and CBD that can help alleviate certain medical conditions, but at what cost? It is still worth looking at for some people who do not require large doses, although it is important to understand the advantages and disadvantages, especially compared to other forms of delivery. It will perhaps always be the delivery method of choice for some people that have been using it for years, but it is unlikely to be the choice for people that are just now deciding to take up medical cannabis.

Advantages:
- Smoking cannabis is one of the fastest delivery methods, taking only seconds to feel the effects.
- Minimal investment in equipment.

Disadvantages:

- Chemicals other than THC can exist in the smoke and be potentially carcinogenic.
- Lung problems can be exacerbated by the inhalation of smoke.
- The smell of cannabis sticks to the room a person is in, the clothes they are wearing, etc.

Using a Vaporizer

For medical cannabis users, a vaporizer is one of the most highly recommended options. By eliminating the need for inhaling smoke, vaporizing can eliminate some problems. The cannabis is heated to around 248 degrees, the temperature at which the active ingredients can be "vaporized," without burning the plant matter itself. There are many different kinds of vaporizers that are currently used, which can help people find the right kind of model for their own particular needs. Most commonly medical cannabis patients used models that plug into the wall and can sit on a table, due to the relatively large size. There are, however, much smaller models that more closely resemble the electronic cigarettes that are now growing in popularity. There are specific advantages and disadvantages to vaporizing nonetheless.

Advantages:
- Much safer for lung function due to the lack of smoke.
- Can be used by people with severe illnesses.
- Rapid delivery that can be felt within just a few minutes of inhaling.
- Virtually no smell when vaporized.

Disadvantages:
- Expensive equipment required.
- Excess plant material is left over and must be disposed of.

Edible Cannabis

The iconic "magic brownies" that many people have enjoyed

before a concert are now being used as a form of delivery for medical cannabis. The cannabis is typically used to create a type of "hash butter," or other fatty food source, that contains the extracted THC. It can then be used to create almost any standard dish that requires butter. The active ingredients in cannabis are fat soluble, which means they can be dissolved into fat, rather than water. That is also why cannabis is detectable in the body for thirty days after use. In fact, as far back as ancient India, people have known that you can blend cannabis with oily foods. In the case of India, it was sautéed in ghee, although made into any fatty food makes it much more efficient than smoking. It is something that should be used with caution, since it can often take up to an hour or more for the effects to kick in.

There is no denying the fact that it is an incredibly effective way of delivering large amounts of cannabis into the system, but there are concerns that many people have, and with good reason.

Advantages:

- Relief lasts for up to six hours after ingesting cannabis through edibles.
- The THC does not have to be inhaled like with smoking or vaporizing.

- Can be used with almost any dish that the patient currently enjoys, whether it is in cookies, brownies, soup, chicken, or even guacamole.

Disadvantages:
- Difficult to dose properly, leading to many people eating too much.
- Delayed effect can take up to one hour to begin, while some people experience a wait of up to two hours.
- Requires a great deal of cannabis to produce, which can become expensive for daily users who require it as a medicine.

Cannabis Oils

It is hard to be more discrete than when using cannabis oils. This also might be one of the most mysterious forms of ingestion for some people, given the unique nature of these kinds of extracts and the kinds of people that typically use them. These cannabis oils are getting a lot of attention for use in children as of late, but there are a lot of people who have found their use is the easiest way of getting cannabis into their system quickly and efficiently.

Hash oil is created by using a combination of carbon dioxide and pressure to reduce cannabis to the essential compounds. This removes plant matter and leaves the user with only the active ingredients that are essential to using cannabis as medicine. This is the most common treatment for children with a particular kind of epilepsy that can be deadly if left untreated. The oil is simply placed inside of the patient's mouth, much like oral solutions for sick children. This is similar to the edible cannabis delivery method, except there is nothing else to slow down the absorption. While many adult patients may prefer to have edible cannabis, oils can be much more precise in their delivery and be much more suited for children.

Advantages:

- Easy delivery for children or people who do not wish to eat foods made with cannabis.
- Easier to dose than edible cannabis products due to the measurable amount.
- Highly effective and high concentrated.
- Affordable considering the amount of cannabis that is used to prepare it.

Disadvantages:

Very high doses are the only way to take in cannabis

oil due to the highly concentrated nature.

- Requires a lot of cannabis to produce.
- The high doses used with cannabis oils have not been studied enough to know the true health concerns that children using them could face.

Cannabinoid Medications

Big Pharma has entered the medical cannabis game, albeit quietly. The introduction of medications like Nabilone and Dronabinol might have not been covered much in the news, but that doesn't take away from the fact that they are essentially synthetic versions of the THC contained in cannabis. This had led to an attempt to have cannabis rescheduled into the same category as its pharmaceutical counterparts, although efforts have been unsuccessful so far. Many people have an interest in cannabis-based medications particularly because they include only the ingredients that have been proven to be effective without producing the signature cannabis "high." In cases where it is difficult to gain permission to use actual marijuana, these chemical compounds can serve as an adequate substitute, but also one that has the ability to be measured more exactly and dosed accurately. These prescription cannabis drugs have been found to have little potential for abuse, however, and they do not feature the signature "high" that other forms of ingestion come with.

Advantages:

- Pharmaceutical grade ingredients ensure quality and consistency.
- Specific doses can be prescribed by a doctor, instead of "as needed" instructions with other forms of medical cannabis.
- No marijuana "high" that comes with many other forms of ingestion.
- FDA Approved for use.

Disadvantages:

- Negative side effects typical of prescription drugs, such as dysphoria,
- Headache, dizziness.
- Rarely prescribed due to scheduling.
- Lack of other cannabinoids that are believed to be responsible for medical properties.
- Potential withdrawal symptoms when ceasing use.

The Battle over Delivery Methods

The medical cannabis argument has taken many forms, but it has also centered on the actual type of ingestion that patients would be using. Most recently this has been the case in states like New Jersey and North Carolina. In New Jersey, the fight has centered over whether or not there would be actual smokable cannabis available or if it would be edible only forms. The law, as it stands, only approves medical marijuana for people under the age of 17, due to the concern for minors smoking medical cannabis. This allows them to have access to the specific oils and edibles that are believed to help with a number of conditions. For people over the age of 17, edible forms are not going to be available.

Leading the charge for edible cannabis have been seniors who are unable to use raw cannabis. They pushed Governor Chris Christie to sign a law allowing adults to use edible cannabis as well, although it was vetoed. In North Carolina it has been the opposite. The Republican Governor of the state recently signed a bill into law that legalized CBD based cannabis oils for use in children with a specific type of epilepsy that can be particularly debilitating and deadly. In this case, the oils will be prescribed by a neurologist as a part of a pilot study to understand the potential effects.

New York state has passed similar laws restricting the type of delivery methods that are going to be allowed. Smoking cannabis would be strictly prohibited. Edible goods, oil extracts, and vaporizers will be allowed for the next seven years as a trial. Gov Cuomo left the option of smokable cannabis open for the future, although it would have to be agreed upon by both the Health Department and State Legislature. In all of these cases, there are disagreements on whether or not these delivery methods are the right choice for the medical cannabis program. Medical cannabis opponents say that states allowing anything other than strictly controlled oils are opening the floodgates to abuse and full blown legalization. On the other side of the argument, proponents of medical cannabis believe that limiting the delivery methods can defeat the purpose in some cases.

This battle over delivery methods continues to show that the argument has many different sides and many aspects that have yet to be worked out. It remains true that the legalization of all delivery methods as a medical cannabis treatment appears to point to an end goal of legalization, making it a more political choice than scientific. Pure scientific evidence has pointed to the benefit of prescription cannabis drugs as well as oil extracts, but scientific research on other forms is much more sparse and conflicting.

That research is something that we will look at in depth in the next chapter. It is an important thing to understand, due to the fact that political talking points often have a louder voice than the actual research studies that are being performed.

Chapter 5: Medical Cannabis: Politics vs Science

The politics of medical cannabis is a very complex and often mysterious part of the movement. Many people have a view of medical cannabis that is influenced more by politics than hard science. This is an understandable thing, though, because the scientific community is often reclusive and quiet in a world where talking points rule the view of the mainstream world. The proven effects of marijuana cannabis cannot be denied in some cases, although many people find that politics more heavily influence their decision. This chapter will analyze a few of the concerns that people have, including logic that everyday people must watch out for in order to stay informed without being influenced.

Medical Marijuana for the Tax Money?

One of the easiest ways of convincing people that medical cannabis is a good idea is by focusing on the potential tax revenue that it could bring in. Colorado has gained a lot of attention lately after bringing in millions of dollars in tax revenue in a short period of time, leading many to believe that this could be a great way for getting their state out of debt that is crippling many different parts of the country. The political arena has focused on the incredible amount of money that the states are missing out on by giving up this market to the black market. It should also be a clue as to whether or not these people are truly concerned about the medical benefits or simply legalizing cannabis and making money off of it. Street dealers of cannabis are not a part of the mainstream economy and they have the ability to charge virtually any price without any real competition. This goes against the tenets of capitalism that America has been built on. With the large profit margin on cannabis, there is a great deal of tax money that is being missed. Marijuana is extremely cheap to produce compared to many other products, although it can be sold for a great deal of money.

Colorado, while having recreational cannabis technically, has a scheme set up that provides the state government with massive amounts of tax revenue. The state charges around 15% at each stage of the process. This means the person producing the cannabis pays taxes, the person brokering deals pays taxes, and the person selling the marijuana pays taxes. For states that are in dire need of income, this is a very enticing proposal.

A Move towards Legalization?

When it comes to medical cannabis, there is always the concern that the politics are actually implying that legalization will not be far behind. For advocates of medical marijuana, recreational cannabis is often seen as in the same arena. With that in mind, it is worth taking a look at what the community thinks about all out legalization. The prime example of this is in Colorado. The state of Colorado legalized medical cannabis in 2000. Even though there was a fair bit of controversy over the coming years, the push for recreational cannabis was not over. In 2012, recreational cannabis was legalized throughout the state. Will this happen in all states that legalize medical cannabis? As early as 2016, many are expecting recreational legalization to no longer be the elephant in the room. At this point, several states could be voting on it, with many of them being states that originally only had medical cannabis. The evidence can be found by simply talking to medical cannabis patients in general. The ones who are saying that cannabis is great for pain and suffering are also saying that it is great for everyone. The mainstream view of cannabis being a harmless substance that can be used as medicine must mean that it is a harmless substance for recreational use as well.

When the time for recreational cannabis initiatives comes, it could very well divide up the people who do not want to deny sick people their medicine with those who simply want to legally get high. By putting them together logically, it can be a much easier sell. Lawmakers in many cases are the people who grew up in the 60s and 70s. They are the ones that enjoyed the recreational cannabis boom of that Golden Era and they would likely enjoy seeing it return to some extent. In fact, several politicians have been arrested for possession of cannabis in the past few years. These are the people from the same generation that introduced American to pot on a large scale. Many medical cannabis patients are older men and women who enjoyed the recreational use to a large degree and have now been able to return to old habits.

An easy survey can be done using a relatively small sample size. This is not meant to be the final say on whether or not medical cannabis advocates have an interest in legalization, but it can give some insight. The vast majority of advocates for medical cannabis have been very vocal about how effective they believe it is for almost any condition known to humanity. Asking these same people for their opinion on recreational cannabis is likely to be met with some sort of support. There is a very small percentage of people who have been supporters of medical cannabis, but have also been strongly against the idea of recreational usage.

The Major Problems

There are problems that no one will be able to get around when it comes to attempts to legalize recreational cannabis. One issue is that medical cannabis dispensaries have in some part been able to use banks. Due to the non-profit nature of their businesses, they have not had many issues. Recreational cannabis stores have not been able to reconcile their differences with the federal government. Even though two states have legalized recreational cannabis, the federal government is no fan of the movement and banks have not been able to accept their money.

In Defense of Medical Cannabis

This is not to say that every person using medical cannabis has a specific agenda in mind to have recreational cannabis legalized. There are many people who have never used cannabis recreationally in their life, but have found relief through medical marijuana. These patients are often very skeptical of legalization efforts and actually take it as an affront to the freedom that they have to treat their own condition with the only medicine that they believe has helped. This is an important distinction before lumping everyone together. The fact remains, however, that at the end of the day, the politics of cannabis come back to ulterior motives, or at the very least logic that could be used by others to convince them that legalization efforts are worthwhile.

But What about the Science?

All of these things could be very convincing to some people. It is easy to show people that there is a lot of benefit to people other than themselves. When someone isn't going to be personally affected by legislation, they are more likely to be in support of it. The scientific community, however, has still been in a contradictory position and scientists and doctors alike continue to be cautious more than supportive. If all a person ever heard was the political talking points, or stories from medical cannabis patients, they would believe that there is an insurmountable amount of evidence pointing to the fact that cannabis is perfectly harmless and that the scientific community is in agreement when it comes to whether or not it should be legalized. In actuality, the science based medicine world has far from made up their mind and they have very important things to say that often go unnoticed by many people. Part of this comes from the belief that the science community has done research that is conclusive and backed up by study after study and published in peer reviewed studies to critical acclaim. The reality is far from the truth. The political view is far from reality due to the fact that there has actually not been as much research as many people would like to believe.

It is easy to point at a single study that showed the benefits of cannabis. For example, one study showed that there was a positive effect on lung tissue when smoking cannabis. This could be a very helpful talking point, but there have not been any studies repeating the process that have found similar results.

The Difficulty of Research

One of the large problems that the scientific community faces as well is the difficulty that they have in gaining the ability to perform research. During the early part of the 20th century, cannabis was still a part of the mainstream medical community. Over time, however, it gained the reputation that it possessed for decades afterwards, in the wake of the Marihuana Tax Act of 1937. The fear of inducing insanity and unsavory behaviors led to the Federal Bureau of Narcotics overruling the American Medical Association and making it virtually impossible to perform research that would have allowed them to make more informed decisions.

This history effectively came to an end in 1942 when it was officially removed from the list of acceptable compounds for medical research. In 1970, it was officially declared as having no medical value at all. With that, scheduling research was put to an end.

The research that has continued in the scientific community has been in a strange place in the eyes of many people. Whereas political movements have focused on the benefits, many research studies have only been funded under the assumed promise of finding negative aspects to confirm federal government regulations. Essentially, cannabis must be studied more before the scientific community is on board with medical cannabis or cannabis legalization, but it is illegal in most cases for people to study it.

Science and Delivery

The delivery methods that were discussed in a previous chapter are often a hint at the political motivations behind the people that are supporting medical cannabis. The scientific world has been working hard to study cannabis in ways that they can, due to the difficulty of researching cannabis. While very little research has been done on smoking or eating cannabis, political advocates tout them as effective ways of delivering cannabis. For the scientific community, however, these are considered very ineffective ways of delivering the active compounds due to the fact that it is almost impossible to measure. This is why the scientific community has been behind THC and CBD based prescription drugs, rather than the raw cannabis forms that many medical cannabis advocates have been behind.

The New York Times once posted a story from an ophthalmologist who discussed what kind of experience his patients had with treatments for glaucoma. He said that the people he was treating would rather not be "stoned" all day in an effort to alleviate some of the symptoms of their disorder. That is why he recommended them take THC based medications, rather than smoking cannabis in order to achieve the same effects. Smoking cannabis four, five, or even six times a day can be very troubling and even bring about many of the negative side effects that people worry about, without providing the same kind of standardized relief that doctors hope for.

The scientific community always prefers accurate dosing as a very important part of treating a disease, so they look down on smoking simply enough cannabis to get rid of the symptoms, something that isn't controlled for quality of can be measured in terms of the actual active compounds that they are taking in. Many advocates believe that the whole plant features a type of synergy that works well with the human body as a combination of different compounds that can provide relief in different ways.

Cannabis is grown by people who may specialize in doing so, but they do not have any control over the specific amounts of ingredients that are in the plant matter. This is a common problem in the "herbalism" movement, as many herbal remedies are not controlled for things like this, leading to problems in the people who are using them. Inconsistencies in potency, purity, or even contaminations from different adulterants can all play a role in the kind of "medicine" that a person is using to treat the condition they have been diagnosed with.

The unscientific way that cannabis strains are marketed can often be of little help when deciding what kind patients should be using as well. There are thousands of different names for strains and the kind of effects that they have could be wide ranging and much different from what the patient expects. For example, many people need a strain that is high in CBD content, but low in THC, in order to treat a condition that responds to that specific compound without giving them a cannabis high that can interfere with their everyday life. When actually testing the strains that have been claimed to be high in CBD, however, many scientists have found that there is very little evidence behind the claims, making these strains simply another kind of cannabis that gets people high, something that the scientific community greatly frowns upon.

Cannabis Politics Vs Science
The battle over medical cannabis is not only between the people involved. It is a constant fight between two major groups that have a large influence over the American people, although one is often heard much more vocally. The scientific community has always had a hard time overcoming mainstream views or political views that people have. It isn't easy to convince people to understand the scientific process, or that they should read scientific journals before making a decision. This kind of fight for the minds of the public isn't likely to end soon, but it can often be an easy task to understand the subtleties when the proper amount of time is taken. The scientific community agrees that there is very little evidence for the vast majority of conditions that medical cannabis is claimed to help. That hasn't stopped legislators from being swayed based on anecdotal evidence that supports a specific position. Policies like these are clearly things that require a great deal of scientific research, although the lack of it hasn't been a problem for many

people. Even more effective have been the stories of people being "persecuted" for their use of medical cannabis. Painting people as victims for simply trying to get help with their medical problems has been a very effective tool that plays on emotions more than science. Whether it is the tax money that entices users, the hope of all out legalization, or the promise of a miracle cure all, political advocates have proven that they have the upper hand due to the nature of scientific research. If the medical cannabis argument was truly based off science instead of politics, there are two things that would have been addressed by now:

Standardization

Having a standardized way of delivering medication is the hallmark of pharmaceutical science, although it is seriously lacking in the realm of medical cannabis. This is why people prefer prescription medications to taking things simply "as needed." This is a major distinction between prescription medication and herbalism that medical cannabis advocates have to overcome.

Comparative Research

It has been found that there is a potential benefit for a variety of conditions, although much of it hasn't been backed up by other studies. It is still important to have cannabis be researched in comparison with existing medications that are on the market. Much of the problem many people in the scientific community have with medical cannabis is that there are other prescriptions available that can accomplish the same thing without many of the health concerns that medical cannabis also brings.

It is clear that medical cannabis is more influenced by politics than science, but there is also big business in the equation. The promise of making a lot of money will convince many people that different things should be legal, and that applies to cannabis. The recent trends in states like Colorado have led many to believing that cannabis is the next gold rush. This push is bringing hundreds of new businesses to the state, investors from all across the country, and many people who have publicly been against the plant in the past are now on its side since there is money to be made. That is precisely why big business is now getting in on the action for medical cannabis. Millions of people are offering millions of dollars to businesses that are selling medical cannabis. It only makes sense that businessmen are now replacing the hippies that many people associate with buying pot.

Chapter 6: Big Business and Medical Cannabis

What has perhaps gotten the most attention when it comes to cannabis is that the business surrounding it has absolutely exploded in the past decade. There has very rarely been a bigger chance to profit on policy changes than this, with many people comparing it to the Gold Rush that hit California almost a hundred years ago. This would seem like a great boom for the economy, due to the fact that millions of dollars are being made, but the problem comes in the form of business decisions getting in the way of medical science, much like politics. This isn't always the case, but it is one thing that should be kept in mind.

Big Business Replaces Big Cartels

One of the popular arguments about legalizing medical cannabis is that the patients should not have to deal with the illegal drug trade. The cartels in particular that bring the drugs up from Mexico. It has recently come out that the Mexican cartels are not complaining about the business that has been taken away from them due to the growth in medical cannabis. There are seven major cartels that have fought for dominance in the United States drug trade. Some have been smaller groups that only act around the border, but the fact remains that they have a large interest in selling drugs to US citizens.

According to the Washington post, the Sinaloa region of Mexico has traditionally been a large source of cannabis agriculture, but they have since stopped planting the crops due to the fact that they are no longer making money off of it. Whereas they were previously making $100 per kilogram, they are now making only around $25 thanks to the lack of demand. A farmer was even quoted as saying that "I wish the Americans would stop with this legalization." The news organization Vice spoke with a retired federal agent who put things into perspective. He stated that there were previously 40 million pounds of cannabis coming in from Mexico each year. The recent trend has effectively put an end to that in large part. An organization that studies this kind of growth and recession shows that the cartels are losing around 30 percent of their revenue to big business.

There is, of course, a conspiracy theory that the government is trying to shut down medical cannabis dispensaries in an effort to help the cartels, although there is not much evidence to support this theory. Regardless of this, it is obvious that there is a lot of money to be made that illegal crime organizations would otherwise be making. When looked at from this perspective, it is hard to argue that business suits would be a much better owner, compared to the murderers that have typically had control of the market.

Non Profit Nature

In order to understand the kind of business that medical cannabis establishments are in, it is important to realize the nonprofit nature of the establishments in several states. In California, dispensaries are not specifically recognized as a part of state law. They are, however, acceptable as a collective or cooperative. There are specific guidelines that they must fall under, but one of them is that it must be a nonprofit. That nonprofit nature has been fairly controversial, since many dispensaries have found creative ways around it. The idea is that the dispensaries are not meant to profit in a big way off this, since it is supposed to be medicine after all. This is often a point of contention since many play up the "community health" aspect of selling medical cannabis, but also post profits of over $1 million a year.

By simply offering other services to customers that are using the dispensary, it is possible to count as a nonprofit without actually worrying about investing profits back into the community. A simple massage table in a dispensary can help them pay their board as much money as possible, while still giving the appearance of acting for the good of their patients rather than their own self interests. This of course isn't true for every single dispensary, although it is something that should be understood when it comes to making decisions about medical cannabis as a business model.

Starting a Medical Cannabis Business

There is not only big business in owning a medical cannabis store, there is also a great deal of money to be made in teaching others to start a business. Seminars across the medical cannabis states have gathered business casual wearing would-be business owners in order to teach them the tricks of the trade, including following the strict regulations that states have in place. At $200 a piece, people can join in on what is a $1 billion plus business. This is an exciting opportunity for people who have probably used quite a bit of cannabis in the past and always wanted to open their own business, but didn't know how to do it. This also opens it up to the world of former pot dealers that are now getting into legitimate business for themselves.

There are 637 dispensaries in Colorado alone. There are also 265 recreational stores now that it is also legal in the state. People are chomping at the bit to get in on this kind of action. There is still a great deal of work that goes into opening a medical cannabis business, with many legal loopholes to jump through, but it can be a worthwhile investment for those that are interested in the business. It is important to keep in mind, though, that the legality is always up in the air, so there is a good chance that it could be a short-lived endeavor once the DEA and FBI raid the business place.

Investors

Investments from certain donors have drastically changed

the way people view cannabis as a part of Big Business. The people investing in cannabis businesses are not at all what people would think. There are no hippie college students saving up their Financial Aid refunds to invest in these companies. Instead, there are stories of people like Republican Assemblyman Steve Katz, a politician who was vehemently opposed to a medical cannabis bill back in 2012. It has come out in the past year, however, that he is going to be investing $10 million in a variety of cannabis-related companies. This is happening through a cannabis investment group called The ArcView Group that is based out of San Francisco.

This investment firm is going to pool millions of dollars together and invest in start-ups that are related to cannabis distribution, security, and software in particular. There are even cannabis stocks that can be purchased by everyday people. Just like investing in any other business, one can purchase stocks in medical cannabis product companies, in addition to investing in partnerships with actual dispensaries.

Will Medical Cannabis Become Just Another Part of Big Pharma?

There has been a major concern when it comes to pharmaceutical companies, especially considering the fact that they are generally seen as being untrustworthy, leading many to medical cannabis in the first place. It turns out Big Pharma is getting in on the action as well, hoping to turn a large profit from a compound that they have been unable to patent. Easton Pharmaceuticals announced recently that they were going to move forward on investments that would cover cannabis growing technology and devices. They see this as a great way to get into the medical cannabis business and ensure quality control that many growers haven't seen until this point. Is this a good idea? There is a great deal of concern over this, especially after they also announced that they were going to be interested in 50/50 partnerships for new dispensaries opening up in California and Colorado. Compared to the overhead costs for other kinds of operations, dispensaries are a great investment for them.

Big Business and Medical Cannabis

This should all serve as a warning if nothing else. Not all businesses are bad things. Capitalism depends on businesses being constantly opened and working in competition. There are still many people that are uncomfortable with the amount of money being made from a substance that is still considered a dangerous thing by many people. The amount of money that these businesses are making cannot be denied, but whether that is a good or a bad thing is up for debate. Many worry that business gets in the way of moral decisions, which is warranted, but when someone is selling a formerly illicit substance there is even more temptation to take advantage of the opportunity.

Chapter 7: The Conclusion

At this point, one thing should be very clear: there is a lot going into the medical cannabis movement. The average American only hears the two opposing voices yelling at each other in most cases. One shouting for their right to use medical cannabis as a treatment for various conditions, while the other is shouting that the patients are nothing but drug users who are looking for a legal way to get high. This can easily stop the truth from getting through. By the time a rare unbiased report comes out an opinion has already been formed. Changing the mind of someone who has already become comfortable with their judgment isn't an easy task, which is why so many people are criticized for being "set in their ways."

MEDICAL CANNABIS

The history of cannabis shows that there have been many peaks and lulls in its use, going far back beyond the founding of the United States. In recent decades, since the research into medical marijuana began, these cycles have increased in pace. In fact, cannabis is actually facing a period of low use, despite what much of the news media reports. Could medical cannabis being widely accepted change that? This is a primary concern that people have across the country. Prescription drug abuse is a very serious concern already, but what would happen if cannabis was just as easily obtained, or even more easily?

The Science

If the science behind medical cannabis backed up every claim that was made about it, it would make sense to see medical cannabis implemented. The risk of abuse would be the same as prescription medications and cannabis would actually be safer than the alternatives that people have turned to in the past. Science has certainly discovered some benefits for users of medical cannabis. As discussed above, many of the benefits do in fact happen, although the problem lies in the other side effects that people can experience.

Does This Rule Out Medical Cannabis?

With this body of research, or lack thereof, it would be easy to say that medical cannabis is something that has absolutely no place in society. Regardless of what the most vocal anti-cannabis activists say, it is possible that new findings could point to a use in the future. Judging off what has been done to this point, medical cannabis can sometimes be effective, although in many cases modern medicine has a better option. Another problem arises with that in mind, due to the fact that research has largely been restricted. Without having some form of cannabis laws changed, it will be difficult to ever know what the true benefits are and whether or not it can be applied to helping patients. Should that research show something as of yet undiscovered, the story could change.

Supporters and Opponents

Overall, it is easy to see why medical cannabis has so many supporters. There are certainly people that have greatly benefited from its use, but whether or not they could be helped in a greater way by traditional medicine is always possible. Both sides have a lot to say. Both sides believe that they are right. The roots of the movement, however, and the research that supports it, appear to be supported by a great deal of political action, rather than scientific accuracy. This is often the case with many journeys, though, as evident by the way that politicians speak to certain groups in an effort to gain their vote. It is plain to see that there is a lot being offered to those who would benefit from medical cannabis legalization. That goes beyond the patients themselves. The owners of the businesses selling the cannabis stand to profit in a big way, often making more than black market drug dealers have in the past. The potential investors can pay off even more for them. All of that revenue also turns into tax dollars that can in turn be used for various projects that local politicians might be interested in, with their own ulterior motives in some cases.

Keep in mind those who aim to legalize cannabis completely. The jaded, hazy eyed pothead is being replaced by grassroots activists who have the discipline and community building power to have an impact on how the world views their favorite drug. For them, medical cannabis is a stepping-stone to making the drug a completely legal substance. This is often a contested point among those in the movement, but it is a common idea that has been raised a number of times throughout the movement.

Taking medical cannabis and removing it from the hands of doctors brings the fear that it will lead to widespread abuse. It is impossible to know if that is the case, but there is far from enough research to know if this would be a beneficial endeavor for the American public. Countries throughout the world have legalized it and seen different side effects, but it is still impossible to know what would happen here. It might not be the end goal of all medical cannabis advocates, although it is an almost inevitable step once the medicinal proponents have their say.

The Final Word

The appeal of political favor, tax money, and potential recreational use of cannabis is enough to convince large groups of people that this would be a good idea, before they have even looked at scientific research into the topic. The uninformed nature of the public at large makes this an easy task for those who would like to legalize the most popular illegal drug that the world has ever known. It is hard to get away from the screaming advocates and opponents. That much cannot be denied. At the end of the day, they are who ultimately decides much of the policy and public opinion that the country deals with. That is true even when they do not have the proper evidence to do so.

The knowledge found here can provide just what is needed for a much more informed opinion. Armed with that, everyday people can have what it takes to vote responsibly and make decisions that could have a large impact on the world. Politics may be running medical cannabis but it doesn't have to be that way. Many issues that are this controversial are typically surrounded with this same kind of enthusiasm from two sides of an argument. It should not be surprising when you consider the entire history of cannabis.

The information in this book hopefully presented an unbiased look at both sides of the medical cannabis situation. There is a lot going on, and a lot in the works for the future, but knowing the facts from the start is important to making an informed opinion.

ABOUT THE AUTHOR

Meredith K. Converse was born to an American mother and an English father in Hong Kong. Since then she has lived in many countries around the world, both for work and for study.

As both a historian and anthropologist, Meredith is fascinated with rituals around the world. She currently lives in South East Asia.

Her motto is "you gotta make your own fun!"

Please leave a review!

Please let me know what you thought of this book, what you liked best about it, and if I can improve this book in any way.

Other books by the same author include:
Probiotics for Beginners
Create Wealth Using the Principles of Feng Shui

MEDICAL CANNABIS

www.ingramcontent.com/pod-product-compliance
Lightning Source LLC
Chambersburg PA
CBHW021411170526
45164CB00002B/598